Nursing Home
Nursing Assistant

Facility
Orientation Guide

Tobin & Associates, Inc.

Richard M. Tobin, LNHA
Peg Tobin, RN

Printed in the United States of America

First Edition, 2019

ISBN: 9781090335494

Contact Information:
Tobin & Associates, Inc.
8233 Howe Industrial Parkway
Canal Winchester, OH 43110
www.tobinway.com

TABLE OF CONTENTS

ACKNOWLEDGEMENTS

William and Christopher Tobin for your support and assistance in the operations of Tobin & Associates, Inc.

To all the associates we have worked with in the Long Term Care Industry.   Every person that has crossed my path has taught me something of value.

Thank you God for your guidance and patience!

INTRODUCTION

This guide has been developed to assist with the orientation of Nursing Assistants to the Nursing Department and all other departments.

To include the Nursing Assistant in a thorough orientation is to make them a knowledgeable and valuable team member.

The Nursing Assistant plays a vital part in the success of a facility and the continued well-being of the residents.

This guide can be used to orient new Nursing Assistants and assist seasoned Nursing Assistants organize their thoughts as they orientate themselves to a new facility, new unit or just help them learn how important they are to the operations of a facility.

One who closes doors to help... limit their doors to opportunity!

Knowledge is one of the cornerstones to the foundation of success!

OBJECTIVE

To assist in the success of the Nursing Assistant in a post-acute setting.

POLICY

This program is designed to provide a complete orientation for the newly hired Nursing Assistant.

RESPONSIBILITY

It is the responsibility of the Director of Nursing to insure that the entire orientation program is completed when a Nursing Assistant is hired.

PROCEDURE

1. The Director of Nurses/ or appointee is to assign a nursing assistant mentor to accompany the new assistant until their orientation program is completed.

2. The Director of Nurses/ or appointee will schedule each Department Director to meet with the newly hired Nurse Assistant and cover (at least) outlined subjects in the Nursing Assistant orientation packet.

    These appointments should be completed within two weeks from the date of hire.

3. Upon Completion of the Area/Specific Nursing Assistant Orientation Program, the entire packet is to be returned to the Human Resources Department of the Area (Regional) or the specific facility office.

EXAMPLE: Schedule of Orientation and Training Program for Nursing Assistants

Day 1
General Orientation _____
Welcome Reception _____
Nursing Administration / Job Expectations _____
Human Resources / Job Description _____
Business Office _____

Day 2
Nursing Programs / Staffing / Schedules _____
Levels of care / Intro to Different Units _____
Risk Management _____
Admission Process _____

Day 3
Quality Validation Program _____
Central Supply _____
Housekeeping / Laundry _____
Maintenance Services _____

Day 4
Computer System _____
MDS / RAI Core Program – Required Documentation _____
Care Plan Process _____
Skin Care Program _____
Restorative Program _____

Day 5
Activities Program _____
Social Services Program _____
Behavior Management Program _____
Resident Concerns Meeting _____
Dietary Services & Programs _____

Subjects to be covered per department/position.
Initial/date each section upon completion.

LAUNDRY	ASSIGNED	INITIAL	DATE
Tour of Department	_____	_____	_____
Flow of Linens / Pick-up and Stock Schedule	_____	_____	_____
Hours of Operation	_____	_____	_____
Lost and Found	_____	_____	_____
Emergency Shortage Situations	_____	_____	_____

Signature of Responsible Party: _____ **Date:** _____

HOUSEKEEPING	ASSIGNED	INITIAL	DATE
Hours of Operation	_____	_____	_____
Trash Pick-up Schedule / Assignment of Duties	_____	_____	_____
Infection Control Process / Bio-hazardous	_____	_____	_____

Signature of Responsible Party: _____ **Date:** _____

MAINTENANCE	ASSIGNED	INITIAL	DATE
Tour of Facility Mechanical Rooms	_____	_____	_____
Gas and Water Shut-off Valves	_____	_____	_____
Fire Safety Program	_____	_____	_____
Emergency Evaluation Program	_____	_____	_____
Emergency Key Storage	_____	_____	_____
Work Order System	_____	_____	_____
Security / Emergency Contact System	_____	_____	_____
CQI Program	_____	_____	_____

Signature of Responsible Party: _____ **Date:** _____

BUSINESS OFFICE	ASSIGNED	INITIAL	DATE
Check Requests	_____	_____	_____
Expense Reports	_____	_____	_____
Emergency Phone List	_____	_____	_____
Ancillary Charges / Billing	_____	_____	_____

Signature of Responsible Party: _____ **Date:** _____

HUMAN RESOURCES	ASSIGNED	INITIAL	DATE
Employee Handbook	_____	_____	_____
Employee Benefits for Nursing Staff	_____	_____	_____
Job Descriptions / Expectations	_____	_____	_____
Disciplinary Procedures	_____	_____	_____
Employee Personnel Files	_____	_____	_____
Payroll / Time Cards	_____	_____	_____
Leave of Absence	_____	_____	_____
FMLA	_____	_____	_____
License Verification	_____	_____	_____
Complaint Process	_____	_____	_____

Signature of Responsible Party: _____ **Date:** _____

ADMISSIONS / MARKETING	ASSIGNED	INITIAL	DATE
Resident and Family Satisfaction Survey	_____	_____	_____
Admission Process for Facility	_____	_____	_____
Notification of Room Assignment / Room Preparation	_____	_____	_____
Admission / Census Meetings	_____	_____	_____
Census Case Mix	_____	_____	_____

Signature of Responsible Party: _____ **Date:** _____

REHABILITATION	ASSIGNED	INITIAL	DATE
Tour of Department	_____	_____	_____
Therapy Services Available	_____	_____	_____
Hours / Days of Operation	_____	_____	_____
Outpatient Therapy Communication	_____	_____	_____
Nursing to Therapy Communication	_____	_____	_____
Routine Therapy / Restorative Therapy	_____	_____	_____
Equipment Available / Requisition for Equipment	_____	_____	_____

Signature of Responsible Party: _____ **Date:** _____

NOTES

SOCIAL SERVICES

	ASSIGNED	INITIAL	DATE
Social Service Role	_____	_____	_____
Behavior Management Program	_____	_____	_____
Missing Property	_____	_____	_____
Resident Concerns	_____	_____	_____
Resident / Family Council	_____	_____	_____
Invites to Care Plan Conference	_____	_____	_____
Discharge Planning	_____	_____	_____

Signature of Responsible Party: _____ **Date:** _____

DIETARY

	ASSIGNED	INITIAL	DATE
Tour of Department	_____	_____	_____
Hours of Operation	_____	_____	_____
Meal Delivery Schedule to the Units	_____	_____	_____
AM/PM Snack Schedule	_____	_____	_____
Different Diets Offered in the Facility	_____	_____	_____
Patient Centered Meal Offerings	_____	_____	_____
Communication Form for Nursing to Dietary	_____	_____	_____
Menus / Alternatives	_____	_____	_____
Orders / Diet Changes	_____	_____	_____

Signature of Responsible Party: _____ **Date:** _____

MDS / RAI / CARE PLAN PROCESS

	ASSIGNED	INITIAL	DATE
Interdisciplinary Care Conference Structure / Schedule	_____	_____	_____
MDS / Change of Condition / OMRA	_____	_____	_____
CMI Score	_____	_____	_____
Discharge Process	_____	_____	_____

Signature of Responsible Party: _____ **Date:** _____

MEDICAL RECORDS | ASSIGNED | INITIAL | DATE

	ASSIGNED	INITIAL	DATE
Order of Chart	_____	_____	_____
P & P Manuals	_____	_____	_____

Signature of Responsible Party: _____ **Date:** _____

ASSISTANT DIRECTOR OF NURSING | ASSIGNED | INITIAL | DATE

	ASSIGNED	INITIAL	DATE
Restraints	_____	_____	_____
Falls	_____	_____	_____
Wounds	_____	_____	_____
Key Indicators (*when due, what is done with information, etc.*)	_____	_____	_____
Skilled Level of Care Weekly Meeting	_____	_____	_____
Rehab and Restorative Programs	_____	_____	_____
Nursing Assistant Assignment Books	_____	_____	_____
24 Hour Report	_____	_____	_____
Basic System / Computer Programs	_____	_____	_____

Signature of Responsible Party: _____ **Date:** _____

STAFFING / SCHEDULE | ASSIGNED | INITIAL | DATE

	ASSIGNED	INITIAL	DATE
Nursing Schedule / Staffing (*Hours, PPD, etc.*)	_____	_____	_____
General Orientation Process of Nursing Personnel	_____	_____	_____
Training Orientation Process of Nursing Personnel	_____	_____	_____
Dress Code of Nursing	_____	_____	_____
Attendance / Tardy Tracking	_____	_____	_____
Nursing Disciplines in Progress	_____	_____	_____
Evaluation Schedule for Nursing Staff	_____	_____	_____
Nursing Assistant In-service Attendance	_____	_____	_____
Compliance Rounds	_____	_____	_____
CQI Programs / Progress of JCAHO / QAPI	_____	_____	_____
Incident Training	_____	_____	_____
Supply Usage Tracking	_____	_____	_____
Procedure for Dealing with Resident Abuse	_____	_____	_____

Signature of Responsible Party: _____ **Date:** _____

NOTES

SKIN MANAGEMENT

	ASSIGNED	INITIAL	DATE
Wound Meetings	_____	_____	_____
Skin Rounds Program	_____	_____	_____

Signature of Responsible Party: _____ **Date:** _____

CENTRAL SUPPLY

	ASSIGNED	INITIAL	DATE
Tour of Department	_____	_____	_____
Central Supply Storage Areas	_____	_____	_____
Stickers / Chargeable	_____	_____	_____
Tracking Forms for Used Supplies / Spend Down Sheets	_____	_____	_____

Signature of Responsible Party: _____ **Date:** _____

ACTIVITIES

	ASSIGNED	INITIAL	DATE
Tour of Department	_____	_____	_____
Hours of Operation	_____	_____	_____
Activities Schedule / Calendar	_____	_____	_____
Community Resources / Volunteer Program and Orientation	_____	_____	_____
Nursing Role in Program Participation / In-room Visits	_____	_____	_____

Signature of Responsible Party: _____ **Date:** _____

ADMINISTRATOR

	ASSIGNED	INITIAL	DATE
Organizational Chart	_____	_____	_____
Corporation Mission Statement	_____	_____	_____

Signature of Responsible Party: _____ **Date:** _____

RISK MANAGER

	ASSIGNED	INITIAL	DATE
Basic Systems / Computer Systems	_____	_____	_____
Quality Validation Program / QAPI	_____	_____	_____
Survey Process	_____	_____	_____
Key Improvement Performance	_____	_____	_____
Corporate Resources	_____	_____	_____

Signature of Responsible Party: _____ **Date:** _____

COMPLETION OF ORIENTATION PROGRAM   DATE REVIEWED

I have a copy of my job description and expectations.   _____

I have established my performance goals and I have my work schedule for
the next month.   _____

I have been taken on a tour of the maintenance, housekeeping and
dietary departments.   _____

I have received a complete orientation of the nursing department and know
the importance of my role in the nursing department.   _____

I have the names of Department Directors.   _____

I know the location of the nursing policy and procedures manuals.   _____

I have an understanding of the CQI Programs, QAPI, Organizational Goals,
Visions and Objectives   _____

Employee Signature: _____ **Date:** _____

Responsible Party: _____ **Date:** _____

Title: _____

Director of Nursing / Appointee Signature: _____

Date: _____

NURSING

Take an inventory of the following: (*check items when located*)

Manuals:

_____ Behavior Intervention and Management Program Manual
_____ Infection Control Manual
_____ Nursing Physical Assessment Manual
_____ Nursing Policy and Procedure Manual
_____ Rehabilitation Nursing Program Manual
_____ Restraint Manual

Suggested Educational Programs:

_____ Infection Prevention and Control for Long Term Care Facilities
_____ Tuberculosis - Long Term Care Facility
_____ Restraint Proper Environment and What About Using a Restraint
_____ Skin Care
_____ Skin Care – Prevention of Pressure Ulcers
_____ Understanding and Managing Difficult Behavior of Nursing Home Residents /
 Antipsychotic Drug Regulations
_____ Resident Assessment and Planning Systems
_____ Care Planning Conferences
_____ Nutritional Risk Tracking
_____ Behavior Intervention Process
_____ Discipline Process